EAT TO DEFEAT FAT AND DISEASES

A Guide to Nourishing Your Body for Optimal Health.

Divine O. Patrick

TABLE OF CONTENTS

Introduction:

Welcome to "Eat to Defeat Fat and Diseases: A Guide to Nourishing Your Body for Optimal Health." In this book, we will explore the powerful connection between nutrition, fat metabolism, and disease prevention. By understanding the impact of our food choices on our bodies, we can unlock the potential to achieve a healthy weight, boost our immune system, and reduce the risk of various diseases.

This book is designed to empower you with the knowledge and practical strategies to make informed dietary decisions that will support your journey toward optimal well-being.

As we journey through, we will discover the remarkable potential of food to be our greatest ally in the fight against diseases. We will explore how specific nutrients and dietary patterns can boost our immune system, support our metabolism, and reduce inflammation—key factors in disease prevention and overall vitality.

Additionally, this book will guide you in making healthier choices by providing practical tips for grocery shopping, meal planning, and incorporating nutrient-dense foods into your daily life. You will gain insights into portion control, mindful eating, and adopting sustainable lifestyle habits that promote long-term health and vitality.

Are you ready to embark on a transformative journey toward a healthier, disease-free life? Let's dive into the world of nutrition, fat metabolism, and disease prevention. Together, we will unlock the power of food and harness its potential to eat to defeat fat and diseases.

Remember, small changes in your diet can yield significant results. Get ready to nourish your body, energize your spirit, and unlock your full potential for vibrant health!

CHAPTER 1

Definition of Body Fat:

Body fat refers to the adipose tissue stored in the body. It is an essential component of our overall body composition and plays various important roles. Body fat is composed of adipocytes (fat cells) that store energy in the form of triglycerides, which can be utilized by the body during times of energy deficit.

Different Types of Body Fat:

a. Subcutaneous Fat:

The most common type of body fat is subcutaneous fat. It is found directly beneath the skin and is typically located in areas such as the thighs, hips, buttocks, and abdomen. Subcutaneous fat serves as a protective cushion and insulation for the body.

b. Visceral Fat:

Visceral fat, also known as intra-abdominal fat, is located deep within the abdominal cavity, surrounding organs such as the liver, intestines, and kidneys. Visceral fat, in contrast to subcutaneous fat, cannot be seen from the outside. It is metabolically active and plays a significant role in metabolic disorders, as its excess accumulation is associated with an increased risk of cardiovascular diseases, type 2 diabetes, and certain cancers.

c. Brown Fat:

Brown fat is a particular kind of fat that burns calories to produce heat. It contains a higher number of mitochondria and iron, giving it a brownish appearance. Brown fat is primarily found in newborns and plays a role in regulating body temperature. It has gained attention as a potential target for weight management and metabolic health.

d. White Fat:

White fat is the predominant type of fat in the body and serves as a major energy storage depot. It contains a single lipid droplet within each adipocyte and is responsible for storing excess calories. White fat also secretes hormones and signaling molecules that influence appetite, insulin sensitivity, and inflammation.

e. Beige Fat:

Beige fat, also known as Brite (brown-in-white) fat, is a transitional type of fat that shares characteristics with both white and brown fat. It is found interspersed within white fat deposits. Beige fat cells can convert stored energy into heat, similar to brown fat. Activating beige fat has been studied for its potential role in combating obesity and improving metabolic health.

Understanding the different types of body fat helps in recognizing their distinct roles and implications for health. While subcutaneous fat primarily functions as an energy reserve and insulation, visceral fat and its associated metabolic effects are of particular concern when it comes to overall health and disease risk.

Health Effects of Excess Body Fat:

Carrying excess body fat, especially visceral fat, can have detrimental effects on health. *Here are some health consequences associated with excess body fat:*

a. Obesity: Excess body fat is a major risk factor for obesity. Obesity increases the risk of various health conditions, including type 2 diabetes, cardiovascular diseases (such as heart disease and stroke), certain types of cancer (such as breast and colon cancer), and respiratory problems.

b. Metabolic Syndrome: Excess body fat, particularly visceral fat, is strongly linked to metabolic syndrome. Metabolic syndrome is a cluster of conditions that includes high blood pressure, high blood sugar levels, abnormal cholesterol levels, and increased waist circumference. It significantly raises the risk of developing type 2 diabetes and cardiovascular diseases.

c. Insulin Resistance: Excess body fat can lead to insulin resistance, a condition in which cells become less responsive to insulin, a hormone that regulates blood sugar levels. Insulin resistance can progress to type 2 diabetes, where blood sugar levels remain chronically elevated, leading to further health complications.

d. Joint Problems and Physical Limitations: Excess body fat puts additional stress on joints, increasing the risk of osteoarthritis and joint pain. It can also limit mobility and affect overall physical function.

e. Psychological and Emotional Impact: Excess body fat can harm mental health and self-esteem. It may contribute to body image issues, depression, anxiety, and social stigma.

Healthy Fat Loss Strategies:

Achieving and maintaining a healthy body fat level involves a holistic approach that combines proper nutrition, regular physical activity, and lifestyle modifications. *Here are some healthy fat-loss strategies:*

a. Calorie Control: Create a moderate calorie deficit by consuming slightly fewer calories than your body needs. This can be achieved through portion control, mindful eating, and choosing nutrient-dense, whole foods.

b. Balanced Diet: Focus on a well-rounded diet that includes lean proteins, whole grains, fruits, vegetables.

Fat Metabolism:

Fat metabolism refers to the processes involved in the storage, breakdown, and utilization of body fat for energy. It is regulated by a complex interplay of hormones, enzymes, and cellular mechanisms. Here are the key steps involved in fat metabolism:

a. Lipogenesis: Lipogenesis is the process of fat storage. When you consume more calories than your body needs for immediate energy, excess calories are converted into triglycerides through a series of biochemical reactions. These triglycerides are then stored in adipocytes (fat cells) throughout the body, primarily in subcutaneous and visceral fat deposits.

b. Lipolysis: Lipolysis is the process of fat breakdown. When your body needs energy, it signals the release of stored triglycerides from fat cells. Hormones like adrenaline and glucagon stimulate lipolysis, and enzymes called lipases break down triglycerides into fatty acids and glycerol. These fatty acids are then transported through the bloodstream to be used as fuel by various tissues, including muscles, liver, and heart.

c. Energy Utilization: Fatty acids derived from lipolysis can be metabolized in the mitochondria of cells to generate ATP, the body's primary energy currency. During periods of intense physical activity or prolonged fasting, fatty acids become a crucial energy source. Balancing lipogenesis and lipolysis is important for maintaining a healthy body fat level. Excess calorie intake and a sedentary lifestyle can lead to increased fat storage while creating an energy deficit through calorie restriction and physical activity can promote fat breakdown and weight loss.

Myths and Misconceptions about Fat:

Myth: All Fat is Bad for You.

Fact: Not all fat is unhealthy. Healthy fats, such as monounsaturated and polyunsaturated fats found in foods like avocados, nuts, seeds, and olive oil, are essential for our bodies and offer numerous health benefits, including supporting heart health and aiding in nutrient absorption. It is trans fats and excessive intake of saturated fats that are associated with negative health effects.

Myth: Eating Fat Makes You Fat.

Fact: While consuming excessive calories from any source can contribute to weight gain, dietary fat itself is not solely responsible for weight gain. Weight management is determined by overall calorie intake, balanced macronutrient consumption, and energy expenditure. Healthy fats can provide satiety, promote hormone balance, and support weight loss when consumed in moderation as part of a balanced diet.

Myth: Low-Fat or Fat-Free Foods Are Always Healthy.

Fact: Many low-fat or fat-free foods often compensate for the reduction in fat by increasing sugar or artificial additives to enhance taste and texture. These products can be high in calories and unhealthy ingredients. Reading labels and choosing whole, unprocessed foods whenever possible is important.

Myth: Fat-Free Diets are the Healthiest.

Fact: Eliminating fat from your diet is not healthy. Fat is necessary for the absorption of fat-soluble vitamins, the production of hormones, and the proper functioning of cells. A well-balanced diet should include a moderate amount of healthy fats to support overall health.

Myth: Spot Reduction of Fat is Possible.

Fact: It's a common misconception that you can target specific areas of your body to reduce fat through exercise or specific diets. In reality, fat loss occurs throughout the body as a result of a calorie deficit and overall weight loss. Incorporating regular exercise and a balanced diet can help reduce overall body fat.

Myth: Eating Fat Increases Cholesterol Levels.

Fact: Dietary cholesterol and saturated fat were once thought to be major contributors to high blood cholesterol levels. However, current research suggests that dietary cholesterol has a limited impact on blood cholesterol levels for most individuals. It is more important to focus on reducing trans fats and consuming a balanced diet to support heart health.

Myth: Eating Fat Leads to Heart Disease.

Fact: While excessive consumption of unhealthy fats can contribute to heart disease, it is not solely the result of consuming dietary fat. Other factors, such as genetics, overall diet quality, physical activity, smoking, and stress, also play significant roles in heart disease development. A balanced diet that includes healthy fats, along with regular exercise and lifestyle modifications, can support heart health.

It is essential to keep in mind that individual dietary requirements and health conditions may differ. It is always recommended to consult with healthcare professionals or registered dietitians for personalized advice based on your specific circumstances. By debunking these myths and understanding the role of fats in a healthy diet, you can make informed choices that support your overall well-being.

CHAPTER 2

How to eat and defeat fat and diseases

To eat well and "defeat fat and diseases" refers to adopting a healthy approach to eating that focuses on nourishing your body, making sustainable choices, and achieving your health goals without feeling restricted or deprived. *Here's an explanation of how to eat well and defeat fat and diseases:*

Listen to Your Body:

a. Mindful Eating: Pay attention to your body's hunger and fullness cues. Eat when you are hungry and stop eating when you are satisfied comfortably.

b. Eat Intuitively: Tune in to your body's needs and preferences. Choose foods that make you feel good and energized, and honor your cravings in moderation.

Choose Nutrient-Dense Foods:

a. Whole Foods: Focus on consuming a variety of whole, minimally processed foods. Incorporate a lot of natural products, vegetables, whole grains, lean proteins, and healthy fats into your diet.

b. Balanced Meals: Aim to create balanced meals that contain a combination of macronutrients (carbohydrates, proteins, and fats) to provide sustained energy and support overall health.

c. Prioritize Nutrients: Make sure to get a wide range of essential nutrients, such as vitamins, minerals, fiber, and antioxidants, through your food choices.

Practice Portion Control:

a. Mindful Portions: Be mindful of portion sizes to avoid overeating. Use visual cues, portion control tools, or measuring cups to guide your serving sizes.

b. Plate Composition: Fill your plate with a variety of colorful vegetables, a portion of lean protein, a serving of whole grains, and a small amount of healthy fats.

Develop Healthy Habits:

a. Cooking at Home: Prepare meals at home using fresh ingredients. This allows you to have control over the ingredients and cooking methods, reducing reliance on processed foods.

b. Meal Planning: Plan your meals and snacks to ensure a well-balanced diet. This can help you make healthier choices and avoid impulsive, less nutritious options.

c. Hydration: Make sure you drink enough water throughout the day to stay hydrated. It supports digestion, metabolism, and overall well-being.

Practice Moderation, Not Deprivation:

a. Enjoy Treats Mindfully: Allow yourself occasional indulgences without guilt. Practice moderation and savor the flavors of your favorite treats, emphasizing balance rather than strict restriction.

b. Nourish, Don't Punish: Instead of viewing food as the enemy, focus on nourishing your body with wholesome foods that provide sustenance and enjoyment.

Seek Support and Guidance:

a. Consult Professionals: Seek guidance from registered dietitians or nutritionists who can provide personalized advice based on your specific health goals and requirements.

b. Community and Accountability: Connect with others who share similar health goals or join supportive communities that provide encouragement, motivation, and helpful tips.

Healthy Eating Habits:

a. Balanced and Varied Diet: Focus on consuming a wide range of nutrient-dense foods, including fruits, vegetables, whole grains, lean proteins, and healthy fats. This provides a diverse array of vitamins, minerals, antioxidants, and other essential nutrients.

b. Colorful Plate: Aim to have a colorful plate with a variety of fruits and vegetables. Different colors indicate different nutrient profiles, so incorporating a rainbow of produce can provide a broad spectrum of health benefits.

c. Reduce Processed Foods: Limit the consumption of processed and packaged foods that are often high in added sugars, unhealthy fats, and artificial additives. When you can, choose whole, unprocessed foods.

d. Hydration: This needs to be emphasised, drink water throughout the day to maintain adequate hydration. Limit sugary beverages and alcohol consumption.

e. Portion Control: Practice portion control to avoid overeating. Pay attention to serving sizes and your body's signals of hunger and fullness.

Disease Prevention Strategies:

a. Weight Management: Maintain a healthy weight through a combination of healthy eating and regular physical activity. This can reduce the risk of various diseases, including heart disease, diabetes, and certain cancers.

b. Physical Activity: Engage in regular exercise to improve cardiovascular health, strengthen muscles and bones, and boost overall well-being. Include a mix of aerobic exercises (such as brisk walking, jogging, or cycling) and strength training activities (such as weightlifting or bodyweight exercises).

c. Regular Health Check-ups: Schedule routine check-ups with your healthcare provider to monitor your health, detect any potential issues early on, and receive necessary screenings and vaccinations.

d. Find Activities You Enjoy: Choose physical activities that you enjoy and that fit your lifestyle. As a result, it's more likely that you'll stay with them in the long run. It could be dancing, swimming, cycling, hiking, or any other activity that gets you moving and raises your heart rate.

e. Incorporate Movement Throughout the Day: Make it a habit to incorporate movement into your daily routine. Take the stairs instead of the elevator, go for short walks during breaks, or do stretching exercises while watching TV.

Disease-Fighting Foods:

a. Antioxidant-Rich Foods: It include foods rich in antioxidants, such as berries, leafy greens, nuts, seeds, and colorful vegetables. Antioxidants help protect the body against cellular damage and inflammation, reducing the risk of chronic diseases.

b. Omega-3 Fatty Acids: Incorporate sources of omega-3 fatty acids, such as fatty fish (salmon, sardines), flaxseeds, chia seeds, and walnuts. Omega-3s have anti-inflammatory properties and support heart and brain health.

c. Fiber-Rich Foods: Consume ample amounts of fiber from sources like whole grains, legumes, fruits, and vegetables. Fiber aids digestion, promotes satiety, regulates blood sugar levels, and supports a healthy gut microbiome.

d. Eating Plant-Based Food: You might want to think about having more meals that are made of plants. Diets that are based on plants have been shown to lower the risk of obesity, heart disease, type 2 diabetes, and some types of cancer.

Regular Health Check-ups:

a. Routine Screenings: Follow recommended guidelines for health screenings and examinations based on your age, sex, and family history. Regular screenings can help detect diseases or conditions at an early stage when they are more manageable.

b. Vaccinations: Stay up to date with vaccinations to protect against infectious diseases. Consult with your healthcare provider to ensure you receive the necessary immunizations for your age and specific health conditions.

c. Health Monitoring: Keep track of your health indicators such as blood pressure, cholesterol levels, blood sugar levels, and body mass index (BMI). Regular monitoring allows you to identify any abnormalities and take appropriate action.

Stress Reduction:

a. Stress Management Techniques: Develop effective stress management techniques to reduce the negative impact of chronic stress on your health. This could include practices such as meditation, deep breathing exercises, yoga, journaling, or engaging in hobbies that help you relax and unwind.

b. Work-Life Balance: Strive for a healthy work-life balance by setting boundaries, prioritizing self-care, and ensuring you have time for activities and relationships that bring you joy and fulfillment.

c. Support System: Build a strong support system of friends, family, or professionals who can provide emotional support and guidance during stressful times. Seeking help when needed can improve your ability to cope with stress and prevent its negative impact on your health.

Revitalize Your Metabolism

"Revitalize Your Metabolism" refers to adopting strategies and lifestyle changes that support a healthy metabolism. Metabolism refers to the complex set of biochemical processes in the body that convert food into energy and perform various other functions. Here are some key factors to consider when aiming to heal and optimize your metabolism:

Balanced and Nutrient-Dense Diet:

a. Eat Regularly: Avoid prolonged periods of fasting and ensure you eat regular meals and snacks throughout the day. This prevents energy crashes and keeps your metabolism active.

b. Include Protein: Consume adequate amounts of protein in your diet. Protein has a higher thermic effect, meaning it requires more energy for digestion and can increase metabolic rate temporarily.

c. Choose Whole Foods: Focus on consuming whole, unprocessed foods that are rich in nutrients. Lean proteins, whole grains, vegetables, and healthy fats are among these. Avoid or limit processed foods, which are often high in added sugars, unhealthy fats, and artificial additives.

d. Stay Hydrated: Drink plenty of water throughout the day. Proper hydration supports optimal metabolic function and helps maintain cellular processes.

Regular Physical Activity:

a. Strength Training: Engage in regular strength training exercises. Building lean muscle mass can increase your basal metabolic rate

(BMR), as muscle tissue requires more energy to maintain than fat tissue.

b. Cardiovascular Exercise: Incorporate aerobic exercises like walking, jogging, swimming, or cycling. Cardiovascular workouts can help burn calories, improve cardiovascular health, and support overall metabolic function.

c. Active Lifestyle: Aim to stay active throughout the day by incorporating non-exercise physical activities, such as taking the stairs, walking or biking instead of driving, and engaging in hobbies or sports.

Adequate Sleep:

Prioritize getting sufficient sleep regularly. Lack of sleep can disrupt hormonal balance, including the hormones that regulate appetite and metabolism. Try to get 7-9 hours of good sleep each night.

Hormonal Balance:

Hormones play a significant role in regulating metabolism. Consult with a healthcare professional if you suspect hormonal imbalances, such as thyroid issues or insulin resistance. Appropriate treatment and management can help restore optimal metabolic function.

Avoid Crash Diets:

Steer clear of restrictive and extreme diets that severely limit calorie intake. While they may lead to short-term weight loss, they can significantly slow down your metabolism over time. Instead, focus on making lifestyle adjustments that are enduring and lasting.

Food for metabolism

Different types of food play important roles in supporting metabolism. *Here's an explanation of each type:*

a. Carbohydrates: Carbohydrates are the body's primary source of energy. There are two main types of carbohydrates:

Simple carbohydrates: These are found in foods like sugar, honey, and fruits. They are quickly digested and can cause rapid spikes in blood sugar levels.

Complex carbohydrates: These are found in foods like whole grains, legumes, and vegetables. They provide a steady release of energy and contain fiber, which aids digestion and promotes feelings of fullness.

b. Proteins: Proteins are essential for building and repairing tissues, producing enzymes and hormones, and supporting various metabolic processes. There are both animal-based and plant-based protein sources:

Animal-based proteins: These include meat, poultry, fish, and dairy products. They supply the body with all of the necessary amino acids.

Plant-based proteins: These include legumes, tofu, tempeh, and quinoa. While they may not provide all essential amino acids individually, combining different plant-based protein sources can ensure a complete amino acid profile.

c. Fats: Fats play a crucial role in metabolism by providing energy, insulating and protecting organs, and aiding in the absorption of fat-soluble vitamins. It's important to focus on healthy fats and limit unhealthy fats:

Healthy fats: These include avocados, nuts, seeds, and olive oil. They contain monounsaturated and polyunsaturated fats, which are beneficial for heart health and overall metabolism.

Unhealthy fats: Trans fats and saturated fats, found in processed and fried foods, should be limited as they can increase the risk of heart disease and negatively impact metabolism.

d. Vitamins and Minerals:

Micronutrients, such as vitamins and minerals, are essential for various metabolic processes. Including a variety of vitamin-rich and mineral-rich foods is important for overall health and metabolism:

Vitamin-rich foods: Citrus fruits, leafy greens, dairy products, and fortified foods are good sources of vitamins like vitamin C, vitamin D, and vitamin B complex.

Mineral-rich foods: Lean meats, seafood, legumes, and nuts provide essential minerals such as iron, zinc, magnesium, and calcium.

When planning meals for metabolism, it's important to focus on balancing macronutrients, spreading meals throughout the day, and considering individual dietary needs and goals. A varied and balanced diet that incorporates these different types of food can support a healthy metabolism and overall well-being.

CHAPTER 3

The body's defense systems against diseases

The human body has remarkable defense mechanisms that work together to protect against diseases and maintain overall health. *Here are some key defense systems:*

Immune System:

a. *Immunity innate:* The body's first line of defense against pathogens is the innate immune system. It includes physical barriers like the skin, mucous membranes, and secretions that prevent the entry of harmful microorganisms. It also involves immune cells, such as neutrophils and macrophages, that engulf and destroy pathogens.

b. *Adaptive Immunity:* The adaptive immune system is a specialized defense mechanism that develops after exposure to specific pathogens. It involves immune cells called lymphocytes, including B cells and T cells, which recognize and respond to specific antigens. Once activated, these cells produce antibodies or directly destroy infected cells, providing long-term protection against specific pathogens.

c. *Lymphatic System:*
The lymphatic system is a network of vessels, organs (such as lymph nodes, spleen, and thymus), and immune cells that work together to fight infections and remove toxins from the body. It helps transport lymph fluid, which contains immune cells and waste products, filtering it through lymph nodes to detect and eliminate pathogens.

d. *Inflammatory Response:*
Inflammation is a vital defense mechanism triggered in response to injury or infection. It involves the release of chemicals, such as cytokines and histamines, which increase blood flow to the affected area and attract immune cells. Inflammation helps isolate and destroy pathogens, remove damaged tissues, and initiate the healing process.

e. *Antimicrobial Substances:*

The body produces various antimicrobial substances that directly inhibit the growth and activity of pathogens. Examples include antimicrobial peptides, enzymes, and chemicals found in bodily secretions like saliva, tears, and mucus. These substances help kill or neutralize pathogens before they can cause harm.

f. Microbiota:

The human body harbors a vast community of beneficial microorganisms, known as the microbiota, primarily in the gut. These microbes play a crucial role in maintaining immune function and overall health. They help train and regulate the immune system, compete with harmful pathogens for resources, and produce substances that inhibit the growth of harmful bacteria.

g. Skin and Mucous Membranes:

The skin acts as a physical barrier, preventing the entry of pathogens. It also produces antimicrobial substances and houses immune cells. Mucous membranes, found in the respiratory, digestive, and reproductive tracts, secrete mucus that traps pathogens and contains antimicrobial components.

h. Fever Response:

When the body detects an infection, it may raise its internal temperature, resulting in a fever. Fever helps create an unfavorable environment for pathogens, as higher body temperatures can inhibit their growth and replication. It also stimulates immune responses and enhances the activity of immune cells.

It's important to note that these defense systems are interconnected and work in harmony to protect the body from diseases. However, maintaining a healthy lifestyle, including proper nutrition, regular exercise, adequate sleep, and stress management, is essential for supporting these defense mechanisms and optimizing overall immune function.

CHAPTER 4

MediterAsian Approach

"MediterAsian" is a term that combines the principles of the Mediterranean diet and Asian cuisine. It represents a fusion of healthy eating patterns from two different regions known for their beneficial effects on overall health and well-being. *Let's explore the key characteristics and benefits of the MediterAsian approach to food:*

Emphasis on Plant-Based Foods:

Both the Mediterranean diet and traditional Asian cuisines heavily rely on plant-based foods. The MediterAsian diet encourages the consumption of a wide variety of fruits, vegetables, legumes, whole grains, and nuts, providing essential vitamins, minerals, antioxidants, and dietary fiber.

Healthy Fats:

Mediterranean cuisine is renowned for its emphasis on healthy fats, primarily in the form of olive oil and nuts. Similarly, Asian cuisines incorporate healthy fats from sources such as avocados, sesame oil, and coconut milk. These fats are rich in monounsaturated and polyunsaturated fats, which have been associated with numerous health benefits, including cardiovascular health and reduced inflammation.

Lean Protein Sources:

The MediterAsian diet promotes the consumption of lean protein sources, such as fish, poultry, tofu, tempeh, and legumes. These proteins are lower in saturated fats compared to red meat, making them a healthier choice for supporting heart health and maintaining a balanced diet.

Seafood Consumption:

Both Mediterranean and Asian diets include a significant amount of seafood, which is rich in omega-3 fatty acids, vitamins, and minerals. Regular consumption of fatty fish like salmon, sardines, and mackerel can provide essential nutrients and contribute to heart health and brain function.

Whole Grains and Complex Carbohydrates:

Whole grains and complex carbohydrates are staples in both the Mediterranean and Asian diets. These include foods like brown rice, quinoa, whole wheat, and various types of noodles. These carbohydrates provide sustained energy, fiber, and a range of nutrients.

Flavorful Herbs and Spices:

Both Mediterranean and Asian cuisines rely on herbs, spices, and aromatic ingredients to enhance flavor without excessive salt or unhealthy additives. Incorporating herbs and spices like basil, oregano, turmeric, ginger, garlic, and lemongrass can add depth to MediterAsian dishes while providing potential health benefits.

The MediterAsian approach emphasizes portion control and moderation. It encourages mindful eating, savoring the flavors and textures of each dish, and being aware of hunger and satiety cues.

The MediterAsian diet offers a diverse range of foods, flavors, and cultural influences. It combines the health-promoting aspects of the Mediterranean diet, known for its association with reduced risk of heart disease, and the traditional Asian diet, associated with benefits like weight management and longevity. By adopting a MediterAsian approach to food, individuals can enjoy a varied and nutrient-rich diet that supports overall health and well-being.

Tips for Grocery Shopping:

Make a List: Before heading to the grocery store, create a list of the items you need. This will help you stay focused and avoid impulsive purchases of unhealthy foods.

Plan Meals in Advance: Plan your meals for the week and create a corresponding shopping list. This will ensure you have all the ingredients you need to prepare nutritious meals and reduce the temptation to buy unhealthy convenience foods.

Shop the Perimeter: The perimeter of the grocery store is typically where fresh produce, lean proteins, and dairy products are located. Focus on filling your cart with these whole, unprocessed foods, as they are generally healthier options.

Read Food Labels: Read food labels and ingredient lists carefully. Look for foods low in sodium, added sugars, and saturated and trans fats. Choose products with simpler, recognizable ingredients.

Fill Your Cart with Color: Aim to incorporate a variety of colorful fruits and vegetables in your shopping cart. These vibrant foods are packed with essential vitamins, minerals, and antioxidants that support your overall health.

Choose Whole Grains: Choose whole grains like quinoa, whole wheat bread, brown rice, and oats. These provide more fiber and nutrients compared to refined grains, which can aid in digestion and help you feel fuller for longer.

Include Lean Proteins: Select lean sources of protein like skinless poultry, fish, tofu, legumes, and low-fat dairy products. These protein sources are lower in saturated fat and can help build and repair tissues in the body.

Limit Processed and Packaged Foods: Minimize the purchase of processed and packaged foods that are often high in added sugars, unhealthy fats, and artificial additives. Instead, opt for whole, unprocessed alternatives whenever possible.

Be Mindful of Portions: Pay attention to portion sizes, especially when buying snacks or pre-packaged meals. Be cautious of oversized packages that can lead to excessive consumption. Opt for single-serving options or portion-out snacks yourself.

Stock up on Healthy Snacks: Fill your pantry with healthy snack options such as nuts, seeds, fresh fruit, and cut-up vegetables. These can help curb cravings and provide nutritious alternatives to unhealthy snack choices.

Don't forget to include water on your grocery list. Staying hydrated is essential for overall health and can help control appetite and support proper bodily functions.

Sample Grocery List

Fresh Produce: Spinach, Broccoli, Bell peppers, Carrots, Apples, Bananas, Berries (strawberries, blueberries, etc.), Oranges, Grapes, Avocado.

Lean Proteins: Chicken breasts, SalmonTofu, Eggs, Greek yogurt, Lentils, Black beans, Chickpeas.

Whole Grains: Quinoa, Brown rice, Whole wheat bread, Oats, Whole grain pasta.

Dairy or Dairy Alternatives: Low-fat milk or plant-based milk (almond, soy, etc.), Greek yogurt, Cottage cheese.
Healthy Fats: Extra virgin olive oil. Almonds, Walnuts, Chia seeds, Flaxseeds, Peanut butter (natural, no added sugar)
Herbs, Spices, and Condiments: Basil, Cilantro, Garlic, Turmeric, Cumin, Sea salt, Black pepper, Dijon mustard, Balsamic vinegar
Other Pantry Staples: Canned tuna or salmon, Low-sodium chicken or vegetable broth, Canned tomatoes, Whole grain cereal, Natural sweeteners (honey, maple syrup), Herbal teas.
Snacks: Mixed nuts, Rice cakes, Hummus, Baby carrots, Celery sticks, Dark chocolate (70% cocoa or higher).
Beverages: Water, Herbal tea, Green tea, Sparkling water (unsweetened).
Frozen Foods: Frozen berries, Frozen vegetables (broccoli, cauliflower, peas, etc.), Frozen fish fillets, Frozen edamame.

sample meal plan for 1 week that focuses on nourishing your body and promoting overall health:

Day 1:
Breakfast: Greek yogurt topped with mixed berries and a sprinkle of chia seeds.
Snack: Sliced cucumber and carrot sticks with hummus.
Lunch: Grilled chicken breast with a side of quinoa and steamed broccoli.
Snack: Handful of almonds.
Dinner: roasted sweet potatoes, sautéed spinach, and baked salmon.
Dessert: Fresh fruit salad.
Day 2:
Breakfast: Almond-milk-cooked oatmeal with sliced bananas and honey drizzled on top.
Snack: Greek yogurt with a teaspoon of peanut butter.
Lunch: Spinach salad with grilled chicken, cherry tomatoes, cucumbers, and a light balsamic dressing.
Snack: Apple slices with almond butter.
Dinner: Whole wheat pasta with tomato sauce, lean ground turkey, and a side of steamed asparagus.

Dessert: Dark chocolate square.
Day 3:
Breakfast: Veggie omelet made with egg whites, spinach, bell peppers, and feta cheese.
Snack: Homemade trail mix with mixed nuts and dried fruits.
Lunch: Quinoa salad with black beans, corn, cherry tomatoes, avocado, and a squeeze of lime.
Snack: Celery sticks with hummus.
Dinner: Stir-fry grilled tofu, colorful vegetables, and brown rice.
Dessert: Greek yogurt parfait with layers of fresh berries and granola.
Day 4:
Breakfast: Poached egg and mashed avocado on whole grain toast.
Snack: Orange slices.
Lunch: Lentil soup served with a mixed green salad on the side.
Snack: Rice cakes with almond butter.
Dinner: quinoa, roasted Brussels sprouts, and grilled chicken breast
Dessert: Slices of baked apple with cinnamon on top
Day 5:
Breakfast: Overnight oats made with rolled oats, almond milk, chia seeds, and sliced peaches.
Snack: Baby carrots with hummus.
Lunch: Spinach and feta stuffed chicken breast with a side of roasted sweet potatoes.
Snack: Mixed nuts.
Dinner: Baked fish fillet with steamed broccoli and quinoa.
Dessert: Berry smoothie made with Greek yogurt and a handful of spinach.
Day 6:
Breakfast: Vegetable scramble made with eggs, spinach, bell peppers, and onions.
Snack: Sliced cucumber with Greek yogurt dip.
Lunch: Grilled shrimp skewers with quinoa salad and grilled zucchini.
Snack: Almond butter on rice cakes.
Dinner: Baked turkey meatballs with whole wheat spaghetti and a side of steamed green beans.
Dessert: Dark chocolate-covered strawberries.

Day 7:
Breakfast: Whole grain pancakes topped with fresh fruit and a drizzle of maple syrup.
Snack: Mixed berries with Greek yogurt.
Lunch: Grilled vegetable wrap with hummus and mixed greens on the side.
Snack: Apple slices with a teaspoon of almond butter.
Dinner: roasted Brussels sprouts and brown rice with baked cod.
Dessert: Fruit salad with a dollop of Greek yogurt.
Feel free to modify the meal plan to accommodate any allergies or intolerances you may have. Also, don't forget to drink plenty of water throughout the day to stay hydrated.
Enjoy the journey of nourishing your body!

CHAPTER 5

Measurement conversions

Understanding measurement conversions can help track progress, set goals, and make informed decisions about your diet, health, and exercise routine. *Here are some common measurement conversions:*

Pounds to Kilograms:

1 pound (lb) = 0.4536 kilograms xtra(kg)

To convert pounds to kilograms, divide the weight in pounds by 2.2046.

Kilograms to Pounds:

1 kilogram (kg) = 2.2046 pounds (lb)

To convert kilograms to pounds, multiply the weight in kilograms by 2.2046.

Inches to Centimeters:

1 inch (in) = 2.54 centimeters (cm)

Simply multiply the length in inches by 2.54 to get centimeters.

Centimeters to Inches:

1 centimeter (cm) = 0.3937 inches (in)

To convert centimeters to inches, divide the length in centimeters by 2.54.

Ounces to Grams:

1 ounce (oz) = 28.3495 grams (g)

Multiply the weight in ounces by 28.3495 to convert it to grams.

Grams to Ounces:

1 gram (g) = 0.0353 ounces (oz)

To convert grams to ounces, divide the weight in grams by 28.3495.

Grams to Calories:

There are approximately 9 calories in one gram of fat.

Body Fat Percentage:

Body fat percentage is often measured using various methods such as skinfold calipers, bioelectrical impedance analysis (BIA), or dual-energy X-ray absorptiometry (DXA). It represents the proportion of body weight that is made up of fat.

Waist Circumference:

Waist circumference is a measurement around the narrowest part of the waist and is used as an indicator of abdominal fat accumulation. It is commonly measured in inches or centimeters.

Body Mass Index (BMI):

BMI is a calculation based on a person's height and weight and is used to estimate body fat. The formula for BMI is the weight (in kilograms) divided by height squared (in meters squared).

It's important to note that while these measurement conversions can provide insights into how fat works and its impact on the body, they are just tools and should be interpreted in conjunction with other factors like overall health, body composition, and individual circumstances.

Macronutrient Ratios:

Carbohydrates: 4 calories are provided by 1 gram of carbohydrates.

Proteins: 4 calories are provided by 1 gram of protein.

Fats: 1 gram of fat provides 9 calories.

Daily Calorie Intake:

Determining or calculating your daily calorie intake is an essential step in managing your weight and maintaining a healthy lifestyle. While individual calorie needs may vary based on factors such as age, gender, activity level, and specific goals, here's a general method to estimate your daily calorie intake:

Determine your Basal Metabolic Rate (BMR): This is the number of calories your body needs to maintain basic bodily functions at rest. The Harris-Benedict equation is commonly used to estimate BMR:

For men: BMR = 66 + (6.23 x weight in pounds) + (12.7 x height in inches) - (6.8 x age in years)

For women: BMR = 655 + (4.35 x weight in pounds) + (4.7 x height in inches) - (4.7 x age in years)

Account for activity level: Multiply your BMR by an activity factor to estimate your Total Daily Energy Expenditure (TDEE). This factor accounts for your activity level throughout the day:

Sedentary (little or no exercise): TDEE = BMR x 1.2

Lightly active (light exercise/sports 1-3 days/week): TDEE = BMR x 1.375

Moderately active (moderate exercise/sports 3-5 days/week): TDEE = BMR x 1.55

Very active (hard exercise/sports 6-7 days/week): TDEE = BMR x 1.725

Extra active (very hard exercise/sports & physical job or 2x training): TDEE = BMR x 1.9

Set a calorie goal: Depending on your weight goals, you can adjust your calorie intake accordingly. Generally, to lose weight, a safe calorie deficit is around 500-1000 calories per day, resulting in a weight loss of about 1-2 pounds per week. To gain weight, you would aim for a calorie surplus.

Keep in mind that these calculations provide estimates, and individual variations exist. It's also essential to listen to your body and adjust your calorie intake based on your progress, hunger levels, and overall well-being.

Serving Sizes:

Understanding serving sizes is crucial for portion control and balancing nutrient intake.

Common conversions include:

1 cup = 240 milliliters (ml)

1 tablespoon (tbsp) = 15 milliliters (ml)

1 teaspoon (tsp) = 5 milliliters (ml)

1 ounce (oz) = 28.35 grams (g)

Glycemic Index:

The effect that carbohydrates have on blood sugar levels is measured by the glycemic index (GI). It compares the rate at which different carbohydrates raise blood sugar levels compared to pure glucose.

Foods with a low GI (55 or less) are digested more slowly, leading to a gradual rise in blood sugar levels.

Foods with a high GI (70 or more) are rapidly digested, causing a quicker rise in blood sugar levels.

Understanding the GI of various foods can help manage blood sugar levels and make informed dietary choices.

Nutrient Requirements:

Different diseases and health conditions may have specific nutrient requirements or restrictions.

Examples include sodium restrictions for hypertension, carbohydrate counting for diabetes, or limited cholesterol intake for heart disease.

Conclusion

In conclusion, "Eat to Defeat Fat and Diseases" is a comprehensive guide that empowers readers to take control of their health and well-being through the transformative power of nutrition. Throughout this book, we have explored the intricate workings of fat metabolism, debunked common myths and misconceptions, and provided evidence-based strategies for disease prevention.

By adopting the principles outlined in this book, you have learned how to make informed dietary choices that nourish your body, boost your metabolism, and support optimal health. You have discovered that eating to defeat fat is not about restrictive diets or quick fixes but rather embracing a balanced and sustainable approach to nutrition.

Beyond fat loss, this book has highlighted the critical role of nutrition in preventing diseases. By understanding the impact of your diet on conditions such as heart disease, diabetes, and immune system disorders, you are equipped with the knowledge to make proactive choices that fortify your body's defenses against these threats. Throughout this journey, you have been encouraged to revitalize your pantry, make mindful grocery choices, and embark on meal planning that prioritizes nutrient-dense foods. By embracing the joy of eating for vitality, you have developed a newfound appreciation for the flavors and nourishment that wholesome ingredients provide.

Remember, the path to defeating fat and diseases is unique to each individual. It's important to listen to your body, adapt your dietary choices based on your needs and goals, and seek guidance from healthcare professionals when necessary. Your health is a lifelong journey, and this book serves as a valuable resource to guide you on that path.

As you close this book, remember that the principles and insights shared within its pages are not meant to be a temporary fix but a lifelong commitment to your well-being. By integrating the knowledge and strategies presented here into your daily life, you are taking proactive steps towards a healthier, happier future.

Now is the time to embrace the power of nutrition, defeat fat, and empower yourself to lead a life of optimal health. Let this book serve as a constant companion and source of inspiration as you continue your journey towards defeating fat and diseases.

May your choices be guided by wisdom, your plate be filled with nourishing foods, and your life be enriched by the vibrant health that awaits you. Remember, you have the power to eat and defeat fat and diseases. The time for transformation is now.

Eat to Defeat Fat and Diseases – Your Path to a Life of Vitality!